Alzheimer's

Been there, Done that!

Now I Am Healed

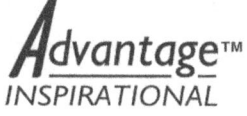
Advantage™
INSPIRATIONAL

Florence Walker

ALZHEIMER'S: Been There Done That! – Now I'm Healed
by Evangelist Florence Walker
Copyright © 2009 by Florence Walker
All Rights Reserved.
ISBN: 1-59755-195-5

Published by: ADVANTAGE BOOKS™
                www.advbookstore.com

This book and parts thereof may not be reproduced in any form, stored in a retrieval system or transmitted in any form by any means (electronic, mechanical, photocopy, recording or otherwise) without prior written permission of the author, except as provided by United States of America copyright law.

Unless otherwise indicated, Bible quotations are taken from the Holy Bible, KING JAMES VERSION, (KJV) which is now public domain.

I have changed some of the names in this book and left out others who are now deceased in order to maintain their privacy and dignity. Besides these changes, this book is based on my life from approximately seven years of age through adulthood and contains only facts known to my family and me and those who were a part of my life.

Library of Congress Control Number: 2009924659

Cover design by Pat Theriault

First Printing: May 2009
09 10 11 12 13 14 15   10 9 8 7 6 5 4 3 2 1
Printed in the United States of America

AUTHOR'S NOTES

This book was written about my personal experience with Alzheimer's disease. I believe that some of the traumatic experiences I suffered and endured from my childhood and on into my adult years were instrumental in promoting this disease. There is absolutely no medical foundation whatsoever for this belief; it is mine and mine alone. However, science has no knowledge of what <u>causes</u> this disease - only how it destroys those who are afflicted with it, what some of its signs are, and the knowledge of those medicines which are being used to give some relief from the suffering.

As one who was afflicted with this disease, but has been healed, I write of those things science could never know. Thank God and Him only, for healing and delivering me. I give Him all the glory.

Florence Walker

DEDICATION

This book is dedicated to the families of the millions of those who show signs of Alzheimer's disease, in the hope that they will no longer allow their loved ones to continue as they are without taking them to have their symptoms diagnosed. I pray this book will so move them that they will not allow their loved ones to be tormented and suffer needlessly any more. They <u>can</u> be healed and delivered. THERE IS HOPE FOR THEM!

The doctors have no cure. While they do offer medicines that are extremely beneficial, they are not a permanent solution. Jesus Christ is the only permanent solution. <u>He can and will heal them</u>. I am living proof of this.

Florence Walker

Table of Contents

AUTHOR'S NOTES 3

DEDICATION 5

Chapter One 9
THE EARLY YEARS

Chapter Two 15
A SHORT PERIOD OF HAPPINESS

Chapter Three 19
UTTER HOPELESSNESS

Chapter Four 23
BEGINNINGS

Chapter Five 29
WHAT ARE THE SIGNS?

Chapter Six 45
MORE SIGNS

Chapter Seven 57
HOPE AT LAST

Florence Walker

Chapter One

THE EARLY YEARS

No one knows the cause of Alzheimer's disease. I believe in some cases, including my own, depression helps to promote it. My preteen years were filled with depression and much unhappiness. I grew up without a father, along with my two sisters. My mother worked very hard to take care of us, but didn't know how to love us (I learned after becoming an adult that she had not been taught how to show love by her mother). I was around seven years old when I heard her say that she didn't want any children. These words hurt me deeply and I never forgot them, for I knew then that my own mother didn't want me and I had no father. I never even knew him. My mother would discipline us by whipping us with an extension cord (many such whippings I well deserved), but there was no love or encouragement shown to offset the discipline. I began to withdraw into myself, playing by myself, and from time to time I acted out the resentment and hurt I felt in rebellion, deliberately disobeying my mother, knowing I would be punished.

I began to block out the memories of those things that hurt me and to lie to myself about things that were happening to me. I would spend days in deep depression, not understanding at that time that I was depressed. I only knew that I was so unhappy and unloved. I wanted someone to help me, but there was no one I could talk to. I would sit down with my paper dolls, which I loved, and talk to them. Ken and Barbie were part of my collection. I always had Ken kissing Barbie, but I became more and more depressed as time passed, because there was no one at home who loved me. I was in a situation I couldn't get out of and there seemed to be no help for me. I was a child, so what could I do?

I loved my sister Debra and we were close to each other, but I never told her what our mother had said about not wanting children. She was eight years younger than I, and I was so glad when she was old enough for me to play with and talk to. Being with her was a happy time in my life. When I was around nine years old, my mother took my sister and I to live with another woman who is now deceased. My mother paid her to take care of us. I don't remember now if she told us why she was taking us to live with this woman, but I remember crying a lot and feeling abandoned.

Even though I had been unhappy at home, it was home and I had been with my mother and sister. Now my life was suddenly completely uprooted; without any warning it was totally torn apart. I began to sink deeper into depression, living with a family who for the most part only tolerated me. I was a source of income, but not loved. Though the lady who took care of us was kind and understanding, I still felt that my life was ruined. I was devastated at that point. I couldn't imagine anything worse that could have happened to me. I was amongst strangers, going to a new school, trying to make new friends, and feeling unloved.

To make matters worse, my sitter's granddaughter, who was about my age, was very unfriendly towards me, even though I tried to win her friendship. So, I began wetting the bed, which I had never done before. I would go to bed at night and not want to get up. This was only because of my circumstances. Eventually, after numerous warnings, my caregiver started whipping me for wetting the bed. This didn't help me emotionally. I began to resent her; but after a few whippings I stopped wetting the bed. Mentally I was in a very bad state and didn't know what to do.

Somewhere along the way, while listening to stories on the radio (there were no television sets then, or they were scarce), I began thinking about committing suicide. Just as television today causes young people to commit violent crimes, the idea was born in my mind to end my young life as I listened to what was taking place on the radio. It was years later that I finally carried out a plan to kill myself by taking a lethal dose of poison. I was about fourteen at the time, but my plan failed.

I can tell you, dear reader, that God's hand was in the plan. He had a plan for my life. I spent many days of my young life crying on the inside, talking to myself and feeling sorry for myself. I felt unloved and abandoned by the person closest to me, my mother. I had no one to talk to about my pain, no one to reach out to. We didn't see our mother. There were no visits or phone calls. She came only to bring gifts at Christmas time, and before the school year started she would bring us something new to wear to school, if she could. During these visits I would cry for her to take me home, but she didn't.

And so it went, month after month. I don't write these things with the intent of painting a bad picture of my mother, for she did all she could to take care of us. And even though she didn't know how to love us, she did the best she knew how to do. I write these things only because I believe they were instrumental in promoting this disease. My mother and I became reconciled after many years passed, and I was able to express some of the despair and feelings that had built up within me over the years. However, I wasn't freed from the hatred which I felt towards her until years later, after I became a born again Christian and acknowledged to myself that I hated her and I no longer wanted to harbor hatred in my heart. I wanted to forgive her because I had learned that if I didn't forgive others, God wouldn't forgive me of my sins and besides, He considers hatred as murder.

I could no longer afford to hold onto the hatred I had towards her. I went to church one Sunday and was given the opportunity to acknowledge my hatred and ask for forgiveness. I was cleansed from it and have been free ever since. I understood some things I hadn't as a child, and asked my mother to forgive me for the trouble I had caused her while growing up. As a result, with the help of the Lord we grew closer and old wounds were healed. She has gone on to be with the Lord, but before her passing I told her many times that I loved her and she said she loved me, too. These were words neither of us had ever spoken to each other before. I was in my early twenties when this occurred.

Florence Walker

Chapter Two

A SHORT PERIOD OF HAPPINESS

As time passed I began to adjust to the new family with which I lived, realizing or believing that my sister and I were never going back home again. We (all the children in the family and I) had jobs we were given to do on weekends. Mine was to clean the bathroom, which I hated. It seemed as though I finally began to fit in, and as far as I knew I was accepted by everyone in the family, except my Big Mama's granddaughter who lived with us. She never accepted me and had no trouble letting me know it. This hurt me because I so wanted her to like me and be my sister. This family became mine, too. I wanted so very much to belong, to be a part. The aunts became my aunts, uncles my uncles and brothers my brothers; but no one became my mother. This never entered into my mind, although I don't know why. I called my caregiver "Big Mama." I also have no idea how this came about. Their way of life became mine.

My Big Mama was nice to me and taught me what was right. She also set a good example for me. She never hollered, fussed, cursed, etc. She was firm and meant business when she said something, but she was a kind, good grandmother. She was a member of a Baptist church and served as an usher there, so we were required to go to church every Sunday and also to young people's meetings. Even though I had no actual training, I liked to sing, so I joined the choir and enjoyed it very much. This became a part of my life, but I still missed being with my mother. I was embracing a new way of life, little by little releasing the old way. I loved the new church we attended, new friends I had met in the choir, and going to choir rehearsal. However, Sunday school, which we were required to attend, was not for me. But we had never belonged to a church before, so I was happy for the first time in a long time.

Big Mama would cook large meals for Christmas and Thanksgiving and other members of her family would come for dinner, bringing dishes with them. I always looked forward to those days. She was a good cook (I think she was born and raised in Mississippi). I loved her greens and cornbread and have found no one who can cook sweet potato pone, a Southern dish, and potato salad the way she did. I learned to make potato salad from her recipe.

I had adjusted to the changes which had so devastated me in the beginning and was excelling in school, looking forward to the events which took place both in school and out and being a part of them. I was never a forward person and was always afraid of trying new things. I lacked confidence in my abilities and myself, but was beginning to come out of my shell, so to speak. I became encouraged to try new things and not be afraid, but my happiness was short-lived.

All too soon, my whole life was torn apart again and I was plunged deep into depression again with no way of escape, no hope. I was a young child with no one to turn to again. As I look back on those days now, I remember it seemed as though everything came crashing down on my head. I was in for another tremendous shock to my young life. Sometimes I just wanted to scream as I went through one ordeal after another. Instead, all the hurt and disappointment was building up inside of me again.

During the time I lived with this family, no one talked voluntarily to me about my mother. However, there was one person in the family who I began to turn to after a few months. I'll call her Deloris. She was my Big Mama's youngest daughter and she was very kind and understanding to me. I would go over to her house to visit and talk to her about what was happening to me concerning my mother and how hurt I was. She always encouraged me, but I was never able to completely empty out to anyone.

My life was pretty stable at this point and for the most part I was happy. During this time no one treated me as an outsider, with the exception of the one granddaughter. I had become reconciled as much as possible to the fact that my mother wasn't coming to see or call my sister and I, except maybe once or twice a year for the holidays or before school started. She would bring whatever she could for us to wear to school. We were really poor, but she did the best she could to take care of us. Then without warning, the thing I never expected to happen, happened, and I felt like my whole world was being destroyed again. I know now it was only by the grace of God that I survived and didn't go insane. One day Big Mama came and told me that my mother was coming to pick us up and take us home, so I was to get my clothes ready.

I remember crying and telling her I didn't want to go. In my mind her home was my home now. I wasn't prepared for anything like this. No one had ever told us that we would only stay with this woman temporarily. I couldn't understand. She was really sad and said there was nothing she could do. However, when my mother came to get us, she tried to make some kind of arrangement with her. I don't remember what it was. She tried to convince my mother to let me stay, but Mama said no. Many things that I am writing now I had no recollection of before - no memory of them at all. Some are painful to me. But because the Lord has healed me, they are coming to me as I write. You may think, dear reader, that that happens to a lot of people, but read on.

Chapter Three

UTTER HOPELESSNESS

As we rode the bus home, I was plunged deeply into depression again. I withdrew within myself. I didn't know how anyone could survive this much pain. Hatred began building up in me. I couldn't think straight. For hours and hours, day after day when I was alone, I would go over these things in my mind and at other times I refused to think about what was happening in my life at all. I would make believe I lived another life. I wasn't functioning normally and part of the time I lived in a make-believe world to escape my pain. My life was a wreck and I couldn't bear to think about it. I would block it out and live a life of pretense to escape reality. I rushed my young life away looking forward only to the day when I would be able to escape, my sixteenth birthday.

Being home again, I never adjusted to my new surroundings for this was no longer home to me. I only endured my situation, passing each day waiting for the next. I must say during this period of my life there was one bright spot, a ray of light in my life, my mother's younger sister, Betty. We called her Bess. She has gone home to be with the Lord now, but in my early years I believe God used her to help me survive. She lived in Chicago, IL and I asked her if I could come to her house during summer vacations. She in turn talked to my mother who said it was okay and I was allowed to stay with her during summer vacation (this took place after she bought a house in Markham, IL). I loved my aunt so much. She was so kind and patient with everyone and I really needed someone like that in my life at that time. She never raised her voice at me or anyone else. She would tell you what was right and leave it up to you to do it.

I remember the pressure and gloom being lifted up off me each year when I would go to her house. She gave me my own room, which I'd never had before. I was so happy, but I still needed someone to talk to. Someone to help me, and I wasn't sure if I could empty out to her. It was during my preteen years that I began unconsciously twisting my hair. I would sit down and for long periods of time, as long as I was sitting I would twist my hair. I would eat my food or read a book with one hand and twist my hair with the other. I have no idea where my thoughts were during these times, but I do know they were not on what I was doing; my mind was a blank. As I said before, many things are coming back to me that before had been lost to me, a total blank. Something would happen, someone would make a noise or say something and I would come back to where I was.

In all those years I didn't realize something was wrong. Only now do I make the connection with the things that gradually happened to me. For years, no one ever said anything to me about what I was doing, until once when I was staying with my Aunt Bess. We were sitting together and I was twisting my hair unconsciously while she was talking to me. All of a sudden she said very quickly, "Stop twisting your hair!" and I jumped. She then laughed and starting talking to me concerning what I had been doing. The only thing I could tell her was that I didn't know why I did it.

I began after that to try to remember not to twist my hair. It took me a while, but finally one day I realized that I no longer twisted my hair. There were times, however, that I would forget, and when I was with my aunt she would remind me. She would always laugh and tell me to stop, but she never fussed at me. Oh, how I loved this precious soul. I believe this was the first sign of this disease because I would be sitting in a room with other people and while they were talking, my mind would be gone. I don't know where, and I wasn't aware it was gone. These incidents were few and far between in the beginning, so I didn't realize that more and more things were happening to me that weren't normal. This is one of the tragedies of this sickness.

So, I continued living this way until I reached my sixteenth birthday, at which time I told my mother I wanted to quit school and get a job. My uncle, "Mr. Banks," had promised to get me a job where he worked and I was going to ride with him every day. This meant that I would need to move in with my aunt and uncle and I was counting on this to help convince my mother to let me move in with them. She did and I was ecstatic. I was finally free. Little did I know what was ahead of me.

Florence Walker

Chapter Four

BEGINNINGS

So, I began a new life again, living with my aunt and uncle in their house in Markham. They had a nice big yard with lots of flowers and a vegetable garden in the backyard. My aunt loved flowers and fresh vegetables; I did too. She would even can some of them. She was a great cook and our meals were feasts to me. We were never able to have meals like that at home because we were too poor. Many times when I was a child we didn't have any food and my mother would try to get us food from somewhere. So, I had my first job, my own money and I was free. I loved living in an area where there was a lot of room between the houses, after living in Chicago where each house or building was close together. You would think I was born and raised in the country; I felt so free and content.

While staying with my aunt I met a young man from Chicago who was interested in me. However, I wasn't interested in him and always tried to get him to talk to a friend of mine that liked him, but he never would. I don't recall how he got my address and I didn't invite him to come see me because I just really didn't like him; but I was seventeen, and had no one in my life.

I was lonely and he was persistent. He would travel all the way from the West Side of Chicago to Markham by bus several times a month just to see me. But you know, no matter how many times I tried to discourage him, he wouldn't give up.

So, after a while, because I was lonely I gave in and we began dating. As time passed I began to care for him and we became intimate. When I turned eighteen I got pregnant with my first child. As far as I knew he wasn't interested in anyone but me; after all, he was the one who had chased after me for months. When I told him I was pregnant, he promised me if he married anyone he would marry me and I believed him. As time passed and I began to show more and more, I noticed he was becoming less affectionate toward me. But this was the type of person he was; he didn't show his feelings a lot, so I didn't suspect anything.

Then one night I went to see him at his house. When I got there, his mother said he wasn't home, so I waited for him as I had done before. Then finally his mother told me that he had eloped and gotten married to someone I knew. There I was, pregnant by a man I didn't care for in the beginning who persisted in going after me and who now had left me without a word to marry someone else. I had seen this happen on television and read about it in books, but never dreamed it would happen to me.

I was alone again and I began crying, feeling betrayed and very hurt. I began withdrawing within myself again, wondering when I would ever be happy.

Foolishly I was looking for the perfect life, a life without unhappiness and pain. I just wanted someone to love me, a life like they showed on television. I was really living in a fantasy world. I asked myself, How much more can I take? As the time drew near for my baby to be born, I stayed at home in bed much of the time pretending I was sick. I didn't want to be left alone again but I was. I was in my seventh month when my aunt came and told me that I had to go home. She didn't say why but I figured it was because she wasn't able to pay for my medical expenses, and besides, she was pregnant with her first child. So I moved back home with my mother so I would be close to the hospital. I remember during the last weeks of my pregnancy I would go to the show by myself and sit for hours, staying at times until the theatre closed, hating to go home. I was so far gone mentally and felt so bad about myself. I had sunk really low and was so disgusted with myself.

My daughter was born in May, but during all this time her daddy never called to ask about her, even though I stayed in touch with his mother. I wanted my baby to know her grandmother. I was so happy with my baby. I really loved her, but this was a love that grew out of my desperation to be loved; it was a sickly love. I would cling to her because I had no one else and would sit for hours holding her and rocking back and forth crying and talking to her, telling her no one loved us, but she was mine and I would take care of her. This was during the time when her daddy didn't ask about her.

Florence Walker

This is a common story now, but back then (fifty years ago) it devastated me. I had grown up without knowing my father, learning after I was grown that he didn't want to know me, and I didn't want that for my daughter; I was determined to give her the love I hadn't been given. There were other incidents after this that I believe contributed to my mental decline and the progression of this disease which I won't go into, some of them to protect my children. I believe enough has been said as to the things in my life that I feel were instrumental in it's promotion of the disease.

It was a few months after my baby was born that someone gave me a book written by the late Mattie B. Poole, a great woman of God through whom He used to work great miracles. It was through reading her book that I learned about being saved and filled with the Holy Spirit. I was so happy. I had never heard about being born again or of the Holy Spirit and had not gone back to church after my sister and I were taken from my Big Mama's house, so those years were forgotten until I began to read my Bible, searching for an answer that I couldn't find anywhere else or in anything else. Then I began to search the scriptures concerning those things that were written in her book. Needless to say I found them in God's Word. When I was twenty-one years old, I accepted Jesus Christ as my Lord and Savior and became a born-again Christian.

I knew from reading my Bible that this was the answer to all my problems, all that I had been searching for all those years. The happiness, love, peace of mind;

everything was in Jesus Christ, in serving Him. As I began to trust Him, I found all the answers to all the problems I had been faced with. It was then that I learned about being healed by Christ through prayer. I have been healed over the years of many things: migraine headaches, tumors, glaucoma, arthritis, blindness and other sicknesses by prayer and faith in Christ. During all these sicknesses I never knew I had been stricken with this terrible disease.

Florence Walker

Chapter Five

WHAT ARE THE SIGNS?

Alzheimer's disease promotes fear and causes a lack of confidence in those stricken with it, as well as doubt in your own capabilities in the early stages. These negative qualities become a part of your makeup and it's very difficult to break free from them, but with God's help you can. Some of the signs known by man are extreme forgetfulness, such as common words or using the wrong words, difficulty with complicated things, major changes in personality, being confused about where you are, becoming violent, suspicious-minded, sudden changes in mood, doing things that don't make sense, etc.

As I write, I will add signs which may not be known as far as I know that I have experienced personally as well as those which are known by man. These experiences may not be in the exact order in which they took place, but they are facts nonetheless. It was somewhere in the seventies that I remember becoming more forgetful, but it wasn't something that I paid attention to at the time. There were times that I was given responsibilities in the church I attended and I would become confused in what I was doing. I had no idea that I wasn't doing my job the right way; as far as I knew it was right. I tried on numerous occasions to carry out my responsibilities only to find out I was doing them wrong. Fear began to grip me whenever I was asked to take charge of some project. I tried to understand what I was to do, but in many things I failed. I wanted to run away, but I stayed praying and crying out to God to help me. He sustained and strengthened me so I was able to go on. He knew my condition though I did not and had a purpose in my suffering through this disease; it was to bring Him glory for He had a time for me to be healed and to be a witness for Him. His purpose was revealed to me even at this moment as I write these lines for I've always wondered why He didn't heal me before, why He allowed me to suffer so long; now I know even as you do. So I became very unsure of myself, not knowing what was wrong. I would have gotten prayer to be healed, but this is one of the effects of this disease. You become delusional and if anyone else other than the elders at the church had told me I wasn't doing things right I wouldn't have accepted what they said. But I believed and trusted them even though I still couldn't understand how I could have been wrong.

In my mind (I remember clearly now) I took time to carefully plan the projects or activities I was to work on, trying to be sure they were right (this happened many times), only to find out they were wrong. Even as I write now, I remember how very traumatic this was for me. I was unable to get things straight in my head, so many things were going wrong for me. I understood very well that they were going wrong; I just couldn't understand why. This is what happens in the early or middle stages - I don't know which it was.

No one knows the torment you endure with this sickness; there were extremely difficult times I experienced as a minister. As I'm writing, I again feel how greatly tormented I was as I struggled day after day to do simple things that I had to do. Many times going to church I would be the first one to get there and I would have to take charge of the service and teach Bible class. Because this was so difficult for me, I ran from doing it by purposely coming to church late, hoping another minister would get there first, but this rarely happened; most times I was the first to arrive.

During this period of the disease, I would forget what someone had said to me right after they spoke. I would remember part of what they'd said but not all and this caused me to panic. Questions would be asked during Bible class and I would struggle trying to remember what had just been said to me, yet I had to continue teaching. This was a work the Lord had given me to do and I couldn't give it up no matter what happened. I couldn't understand, since the Lord knew what was happening to me, why He didn't release me from this responsibility. I struggled to keep from breaking down and to keep from crying. No one knew the mental battle I was having. Many times in my spirit I wanted to give up because I was in anguish so much of the time, but I continued to look to the Lord and to trust in Him, each day being encouraged.

Florence Walker

During what I call the middle stages, my preaching ministry began to deteriorate also. We were taught as ministers to write down the sermons that were given to us by the Lord, and to keep them until the time came to preach those sermons. This I did, but as time went by I noticed my sermons had changed. I had forgotten about the books in which I had recorded earlier messages; I hadn't thought of them for years. I only knew something was wrong with my sermons, but just couldn't figure out what. It became difficult for me to preach with a written sermon as well as without one. How can you preach when you forget what you're going to say?

I was so afraid each time I was to bring the message. This is a great responsibility, because the people must be given the correct Word of God. They have to be edified and this was a tremendous responsibility that I didn't take lightly. Again, I wondered how could the Lord allow me to continue to go through this knowing I was in a bad way mentally but still I said nothing to anyone. My confidence was gone but I continued studying, getting confused but trying my best to understand, as well as remember what I'd just read. As fast as I would read one line and go to the next I would forget what I had just read and have to go over the line again in desperation. Finally I would just pray to the Lord and ask Him to help me to remember and retain what I'd just read and then I would close my Bible.

In the beginning of this disease or my first recollection of something being wrong with me, I could remember the scriptures and quote them, but as the years passed I found that I was forgetting God's Word little by little. I knew I was forgetting more and more but it really threw me when I realized that I was forgetting God's Word. This was something I never expected, never anticipated because His Word is so vital to me in everything. This really terrified me more than anything because I knew it was His Word that saves and keeps you. You must live by it and use it. I knew that if I couldn't remember it I couldn't do it. God's Word is so vitally important to everyone who wants to live for Him. This was where I got my help, where I found answers to problems in my daily life; this was how I learned to live right, as He wanted me to live.

If the Bible were taken away from me I would still be all right, but if I couldn't remember what it said (and this was slowly taking place), I would be lost because I wouldn't know what to do. This was my reasoning. I didn't tell anyone about this, as always I turned to God in prayer trying to stay calm. These were very trying times for me. Just to make it from one day to the next sometimes seemed to take everything I had, but again the Lord both encouraged and strengthened me through His Word, letting me know He had written His Word in my heart (Hebrews 8:10), so I knew I would always have His Word with me even if I forgot it at the time.

Recently, after the Lord healed me, I was going through my books in which I had written my sermons years ago and I was shocked at the difference in the messages I recorded in later years from those written before this disease began to progress. The earlier sermons were more dynamic and powerful; the latter ones were gibberish (this of course was natural considering what was wrong with me) but I was shocked at the difference nonetheless. The scriptures didn't coincide with my subjects and my subjects were like nothing. That's the best way I can describe it; it just was not together at all. I remember how I struggled through the years trying to find a subject for the scriptures I had and was unable to; I just couldn't connect the scriptures together. I still have most of the sermons I recorded (the outlines) now and as I write new sermons, I see a big difference.

This was a horrible time in my life, but I turned to God in prayer for I was beginning to wonder if I was losing my mind; yet I didn't (and wasn't mentally able to) talk to anyone and ask for help. As I said before, this happened many times in different relations I had, but these incidents weren't close together. I never made the connection because I would forget that it had happened. I believe I was in the middle stages of this disease at this time, for I was beyond just forgetting things or repeating them. My thinking had become very slow and I wasn't able to grasp what people were saying to me, especially when they talked fast; without my realizing it, my thinking had changed drastically. I had gone through an identity crisis. I don't know even at this point how I used to be, how I really was, what I was about in reality. I remember praying about this before I was healed and telling the Lord this and asking Him to help me.

There are memories, which have come back, regarding my aspirations to become an executive secretary; I really wanted to work in an office and do secretarial work. I would have been very good in this field but the memory of this desire was gone completely.

Recently my oldest daughter was talking to me about my son and how sick he had been as a child; at first I didn't remember and felt so bad about it. I thought, how could I not remember something so serious about my own child, but while she was talking to me bits and pieces of this incident came back to me and I remembered.

There are no such remembrances while you are suffering with this disease, no vague recollections, absolutely nothing. There have been numerous times over the years when I tried so hard to recall things that others were trying to get me to remember and all there was, was a terrible emptiness in my mind. Mere words cannot explain what this felt like and it is a terrifying experience, something no one wants to go through. Think about it, all your life there are thoughts and memories coming to you, some with effort, some not, and no matter how hard you try you can't remember familiar things. Worse than that is the absolute emptiness in your brain; even now I cringe and shudder as I think about it; it's no fun. I don't know how anyone feels who has gone insane, nor do I want to, but if it's anything like what I experienced with that disease, my heart goes out to him or her. I really don't want to think about these things, but I must in order to write this book.

Florence Walker

I remember saying to myself, "Oh, my God, what is wrong with me?" and then the experience I'd just had would silently slip away from me without my ever knowing I'd had it. Oh, dear reader, if you have a loved one stricken with this disease, I hope this book will convey to you the terror and helplessness of it and will stir up compassion within you for them. "There but for the grace of God go I," is a true saying for everyone who has not been stricken with Alzheimer's, but I thank God for Jesus Christ who heals every sickness and every disease.

I became unable to make quick decisions and it was very difficult for me to hold my thoughts together. I wasn't able to focus on anything, which really frightened me, but I continued to hold onto God, knowing my help was in Him and that somehow, some way I was going to make it. I know that if I had ever let go of my faith in God, I would have been lost like so many others. I remember once when our late Bishop, whom I will call "Bishop Wallace," was talking to me and began to question me about something I had done and I was unable to give him an immediate answer. I was trying to get it together in my head, but as I didn't say anything he began to pressure me for an answer.

This was the first time that I remember this happening to me, but it wasn't the last time; it was only the beginning. As he pressed me for an answer, I flared up and shouted at him. I wasn't sure what the answer was to his question concerning what I had done, but my reaction was to shout at him, which I'd never done before to him or anyone else. I respected him in the position that he held. My reaction under pressure was totally involuntary and I remember thinking to myself again "Oh, my God, why did I do that? I didn't mean to. What's happening to me?"

So I began doing and saying things that were totally uncharacteristic of me. There were times when I would be talking to someone and I would have in my mind what I was going to say, and while I was speaking something else totally different would come out of my mouth, and this too was completely involuntary. In this stage of the disease I still realized that I was doing things that I didn't intend to do but didn't understand why. I was becoming more and more afraid all the while fighting against the thoughts that I was going insane, yet refusing to let fear overcome me. More and more I began doing things that didn't make sense and wondering why I did them, and people began to laugh and make fun of me though I didn't know it at the time. Years later my youngest daughter informed me of this at which time she acknowledged that she too had laughed at me.

But no one tried to help me after seeing the difference in the way I was acting. I was reaching out for help but no one understood and none of my children realized that I needed help; but now I know that it wasn't for anyone to help me at that time because the Lord had a set time, as I said before, for my deliverance.

I had reached the stage where familiar things were no longer remembered. There are things even now concerning my children's childhoods that I don't remember, such as the day that my oldest daughter graduated from high school. I couldn't remember if I was there or what happened during that time. I had forgotten my mother's and both of my sisters' birthdays and had to write them down. I thought at first this was from age and getting older and that many were making this same mistake.

Then there was the year of accidents; this was a time of terror for me because again I couldn't understand what was happening to me. I lived more and more in a state of confusion now, unable to reason why there was so much chaos in my life. I began losing my sense of judgment. I started driving when I was twenty-eight years old and had been driving for a while with no such incidents as this. My driving record was good, but at this stage I couldn't remember directions from one moment to the next and suddenly I was having all these minor accidents one after the other because my judgment was off, although I didn't realize it at the time. There were so many incidents where I was leaving a parking space and no matter what I did, I would back into or scrape someone's car despite how careful I was. I would get out of my car to check out the damage and sometimes leave a note with my name and number so the owner could contact me; thank God my husband had good insurance.

Since I always backed up slowly, most times there was just a little scratch and sometimes nothing that I could see. There were, I believe, at least a couple of times when I didn't leave a note (this was happening so often to me). I was so shaken by these accidents.

On one or two occasions I did dent a couple of cars where the owners did call and we had to have their cars repaired. I was so badly shaken by the last thing that happened to me that year while driving that I almost gave up driving completely. I don't recall all the details, but while driving by myself I almost sideswiped a car that was parked and there was no logical explanation for this because no one was along side me or behind me. I almost lost control of the car trying to keep from hitting this vehicle. I was so scared that I didn't want to drive home and told myself that I didn't want to drive anymore and almost called my husband to come and get me, but the Lord spoke to me and told me if I didn't get in my car and keep driving I would never drive again.

After hearing the voice of the Lord, I realized I couldn't give up because there were too many things that I needed to do for myself. I couldn't see myself having anyone take me around; but most of all if I quit I would be a loser and fear would have won out over me. I felt I had been a loser all my life, and I wanted that to change. I also remembered the saying "A winner never quits and a quitter never wins" and I wanted to be a winner. So I grabbed a hold of faith, believing and confessing that I could do it, and after waiting in the car until I was calm enough, I drove home shaken from my experience but able to go a little further. It was a struggle for me, but again I turned to the Lord in prayer, asking Him to help me, and even though it was difficult,

I made it, and the Lord helped me because after this incident I never had any more near misses or scraped another car during this period.

Let me emphasize, dear reader, familiar things and people do not disappear all at once. There are incidents that take place one by one, things you forget and at first they come back to you. This happens over a period of months once it starts, not years, and then that familiar memory which you've had for years silently without any indication or warning slips away from you; it's gone never to come back, at least not by any man's effort, only through Jesus Christ who heals all who come to Him. I thank God He didn't allow me to suffer with this disease to the point where I didn't know my children or siblings. I did, however, forget cousins and their names, and I had begun to call my oldest daughter by the youngest one's name and vice versa. No matter how hard I would try to remember things, there was always this deadness, this emptiness in my mind, which was a horrible experience and one that will cause you to panic; thank God it's over.

There are many terrifying things that happen to those stricken with this disease. I had reached the stage that as someone was speaking to me I heard his or her words, but by the time it reached my brain I heard something different, even though they were standing close to me. It was approximately the year 2000 when I had my first experience in this area. Our late Bishop Wallace had given me another project to work on for our church and I had completed all that I was to do up to that point, so I went to see him and give him my report. As I spoke with him he asked me if I had done something concerning the report (at this point I don't remember what the question was, I only remember that this happened). I remember answering him and saying, "Do you mean?" and repeated what I thought he'd said and he said no. He then repeated the same question to me over again; I was standing directly in front of him and heard his words but didn't comprehend them.

By this time I was anxious because I knew something was happening to me, but again I couldn't understand what or why. He did repeat the question to me and I paid very close attention to him to make sure I would understand this time, but I still didn't. Bishop was a great man of God and the Lord had worked many miracles through him, yet at this time when I really needed prayer I couldn't ask for it; instead I said out loud, "What's wrong that I can't understand what he's saying to me?" At this point, to calm me, he told me to sit down and began to talk to me, but not about what happened. I never asked him about it, but I believe the Lord let him know what was wrong with me. As we sat and talked, I did come to understand what he was saying and so this incident passed over and after a short time the memory of this was gone, too.

I am a missionary as well as an evangelist and as such, the Lord spoke to me and told me to go to Oak Forest Hospital in Oak Forest, IL, to visit the sick there; this was the work He commissioned me to do. This is a huge hospital and since by this time I couldn't remember directions from one moment to the next, I was faced with the fear of getting lost. However, I had enough forethought to plan how I would go so I wouldn't get lost. I would always park my car in the same lot and try to get a space directly across from the entrance where I would go in; each entrance had the letter over the door for that building and I made sure to go in the same building all the time, after nearly getting lost my first few times visiting there. Each building opens into the next and there were no doors inside connecting one building to another until the buildings changed direction. So, I would go straight through each ward, which was on both sides of the building.

When I had finished my ministry praying for those who wanted prayer, I would continue by visiting with others. It was so tragic to see the many patients that had been placed there and left alone to die with no one to come see them and no hope of ever leaving. After I finished my ministry, I would always turn around and go straight back the way I had come in with no problem. These buildings were long and sometimes I would go to the second floor to minister to those patients. I would come down and go straight out because as long as I didn't make any turns I was fine. This I did for maybe two years, once a week whenever I could. I had become very familiar with the buildings and parking area so I was no longer afraid of getting lost. If it had been just a matter of my forgetting directions I would have been fine, but this wasn't the case and I had developed a false sense of confidence, so I began to increase the area of my ministry so I could visit with more patients.

Then, one day as I turned and was getting ready to go home, without any warning I felt something take place in my brain. It was a weird feeling and something that never had happened to me before. The only way to describe it is to say it's like you're wearing a hat on your head and suddenly and very quickly a strong wind snatches it from your head like "swoop," and the memory of how to get out of that hospital was gone, taken from me. I felt it leave. I stood there near the doorway of the ward I had been in, so frightened that I couldn't think straight. I remember saying to myself, "I don't know how to get out of here." I was terrified of being lost and because my memory had left me in that way. I knew what had just happened to me, but not how it had happened. I had never heard of anything like that happening to anyone and at that time I had no idea what this disease could do to you because there was little said about it, if anything at all.

So, I stood still trying to get my bearings, trying to remember how to get out and becoming very confused. There were people there, nurses to ask, but I didn't realize that was all I had to do because I was still unable to think clearly. It was daytime and at first nothing was familiar to me. In the beginning I wasn't physically able to move. I can't explain why, but I was so terrified and lost. However, I began slowly moving forward. I began to gradually remember how to get out of there; yet there was this feeling inside of me that let me know I couldn't act quickly in any way or the memory of how to get out of there would leave me again.

It was like I became almost immobile, so I moved very slowly and was so shaken by this experience that I was trembling. This was not a natural forgetfulness - it was extreme forgetfulness, where at times you feel something taking place in your brain and I never want to have that experience again. Why is it that you don't have presence of mind to ask for help? I don't know, but for me it never came until I learned what was wrong with me. My anxieties became stronger, uncertainties in many ways increased, and I lacked confidence more and more in knowing what was true, real and not real, what was right.

Chapter Six

MORE SIGNS

Oh, dear reader, if only words could convey to you the horror of this sickness of the mind, but words can't do it justice. Bits and pieces of my life slowly and silently slipped away from me. I went on about my daily life never knowing they were gone. Anyone who didn't know me, talking with me from time to time never knew that some of the things I said and did weren't right. I seemed normal to them and it appeared that I knew what I was talking about, but more and more I recognized that I didn't know what I was saying. I see this happening even now with others I come in contact with. How many people, dear reader, have you held conversations with that seemed perfectly normal, what they said made sense to you, yet they themselves had no idea what they were talking about? You will never know; it's very real to them but it is not reality. This is just how it is.

None of my children knew, though I remember reaching out to my son for help as I told him something was happening to me - that something was wrong with me. He, however, didn't respond. I don't think he knew what to do or say. Recently as I was telling my oldest daughter of how I had been healed of this disease, she told me she remembered years ago that I was doing things out of character and she said to herself, "Where is my mama? This isn't my mama," but she didn't know how to help me because she was so young at the time.

Many are doing this even now. Please don't make this mistake. Pay attention to the signs. If your loved ones are acting out of character and manifest the signs, take them to a doctor and then take them to "THE DOCTOR" Jesus Christ to be healed, since a doctor can only diagnose their case.

As this disease progressed, many times as I held conversations with others, in the middle of our conversation, sometimes even in the beginning, I would forget what I was talking about or what I was going to say and it wouldn't come back to me. Simple words I had known all my life were gone from my memory. I had at one time excelled in spelling and English, but I was at the point where I couldn't remember simple words, and this was happening more and more. Holding conversations became more difficult as I couldn't remember words to express what I wanted to say, and so I began not to talk from time to time because I was so embarrassed.

Now I was at the stage in this disease that almost all the time when others would talk to me I couldn't remember what they said even while they were speaking. I would try very hard to remember but I couldn't and I didn't want them to know that I didn't know what they had said. This is the way it was and it would cause me to panic when what was being said was of importance. Many times because what I couldn't remember was of a business nature, I would have to go back and ask what they'd said to me. On many occasions while I was seeking information for something important, I would try to write down what was being said to me but I never was able to record all the information given to me and I would have to ask them to go over what they'd said that I'd missed. May God richly bless those souls, everyone that was so patient and understanding with me. They'll never know how grateful I am to them for their kindness and help.

There were many times as I was traveling locally I would ask for directions to get to an address; I would listen to the directions given me, but by the time I got to my car to write them down, they would be gone, so I would stop and ask someone else. For a number of years I didn't drive to places that weren't familiar to me, for fear of getting lost. And then I began to take control of my life in this area, but only by the grace of God, because the Bible says that *"...the fearful and unbelieving... shall have their part in the lake which burneth with fire and brimstone..." (Revelation 21:8),* so I was determined to overcome this fear.

I am not one to be cast into the lake of fire, which the Bible definitely speaks of. You ask me, do I believe this? Yes, dear reader, I believe every Word of God. So I took hold of faith and trusted in the Lord not to let me get lost, and I asked for directions over and over to get to and from places unfamiliar to me, and the Lord never let me get lost. There are many that have this disease that have wandered away from their families never to be heard from again. I know of one precious soul personally, my oldest child's grandmother on her father's side. Many years ago while living with her son, they were careless and left the door unlocked and unknown to them she left the house and was never seen again. She was in the advanced stages of Alzheimer's. Her family knew she had this disease but became careless.

Then there was my own mother who lived with my niece while stricken with this disease and through someone's carelessness the door to the house was left unlocked. Not being properly supervised, she walked out the door into a city she had lived in for years and couldn't find her way back home. She didn't know where she was going, but thank God, the disease had not progressed to the stage where she wasn't able to think clearly at all. She asked a lady on the street if she would help her and this kind soul took her back home; she could have been lost forever without our ever knowing what became of her. I believe now that some of the kindnesses I have shown to so many others who couldn't help themselves came back to my mom. Thank God for Jesus Christ!

I love gospel music as well as some of the contemporary music, and many of the old hymns I learned years ago and sang as I took charge of the service at my church started to slip away from me gradually. I would stand before the congregation trying to remember them and I couldn't, so every Sunday I would sing the same songs. Even when I would try to use the songbooks, I became unable to get the lyrics together. These all were very trying and difficult times for me and yet I was still up before the public. The horror of it is that you don't know that things are slipping away from you, and you never realize that they are gone. It's as though you never had the knowledge or memories of those things, as though they were never a part of your life at all. They are wiped out and it's as though everything about you and your life is slowly and quietly disappearing for good, as though you are being wiped out. I cannot express it more directly than that.

I remember a video I bought entitled "The Net," in which the female star played the role of a computer expert who was thought to have gotten some information about a plan to murder someone rich who was in the Internet business. They hired assassins to go after her, and through the Internet they wiped out and totally erased her identity, driver's license, the home she lived in, the car she owned, her passport and even her name; everything was taken from her. When she found out, even her bank accounts were gone. This is how Alzheimer's works. The only difference is that you don't wake up and find that they are gone, you never wake up from this nightmare, not by or of yourself or any other human being.

I began each night before going to bed to write down everything I had to do the next day - from praying to brushing my teeth, washing up, going to work, appointments, yes, dear reader, everything. I dated the reminder so I would know what day it was for and put it in my purse. Then slowly I'd forget to write or read it the next day, until this too was gone from my memory. It was during this very difficult and stressful time that I fought against the thought that I was going insane, again using what I have been taught in God's Word against this fear, that the Lord spoke to me and said, "You have a strong mind, a powerful mind." I remembered His Word, "For God hath not given us the spirit of fear; but of power, and of love, and of a sound mind" (II Timothy 1:7). So, I held onto what the Lord had said to me with all my might. My life depended on my faith in what He had just spoken to me and upon His written Word. So I clung to them, grateful to God for His Word, which encouraged me.

From then on, whenever fear of going insane would try to enter my mind, I fought against it with those Words He had given me. I refused to believe or accept anything else, for God does not lie, and I knew if He said I had a strong and powerful mind, I had it, no matter how things looked to the contrary; this is faith. I stood on His Word. No one will ever know how happy I was that the Lord had spoken to me. I gained more strength to go on, and from then on I said what the Lord said about my mind and I believed it. If I had allowed myself to believe or to confess I was going insane, I would be crazy today; only He sustained me.

In the seventies I began doing volunteer work as a caregiver. This was a gift given to me by the Lord, caring for seniors, which I have now become myself. I wanted to be a help to them, to show them that with God's help, they could become independent again. I had learned not to give in to sickness and infirmities but to trust in God. I carried this message with me on my jobs, and because of this I was able to help some of them become independent again. After working a few short years volunteering, I began working professionally for healthcare agencies.

There were periods between the drastic incidents that occurred, which I believe signaled new levels this disease had reached, that I was becoming more and more forgetful. During the years I worked as a caregiver, about 23 in all, I had not had any professional training; I learned by experience. I would ask the nurses, doctors, physical therapists and nurse's aides questions, so I could learn everything about nursing and in-home care. I never worked on a case just for the money; my interest was in helping those I took care of, so I learned a great deal, going out of my way to help them. Consequently I was assigned cases that were supposed to go to CNAs, (Certified Nurses Assistants) which I was not. After working a few years it came to me, "Why should you work for them when you can have your own business?" I was so excited because I had learned so much over the years. I'd never thought about starting my own business, but I believed I could do it.

I had access to my patients' contracts from the agencies I worked for, so I read them to learn what their terms were for the clients. I had all the paper work my employees would need and I asked my patients questions for all the other information that I needed. I was familiar with everything the CNAs, companions and home health aides needed to know and do, having worked in those capacities myself. There was only one thing left. I had to find out how to get into this field, so I asked my boss and was so happy because he told me how to do it. I went through the process of finding out how to write a plan to present to financial institutions and sent for papers from the Small Business Administration. I gathered all the materials I needed, chose a name for my business and did everything I knew to do except going to a financial institution for a loan, but I was ready to take that step.

Then without warning, silently the memory of all my plans for my own business were wiped out - gone without my knowing it. I had absolutely no memory of it or of all the plans I had made and recorded. So, I continued working for the agency, taking care of patients in their homes until I retired. It wasn't until years later after I was healed that I came upon all the paperwork for my business; and I remembered all my preparations and work and plans. It's strange to me how I took care of so many patients and recognized the symptoms of those with Alzheimer's disease, but not my own.

There were three patients of mine that had been stricken with Alzheimer's from whom I learned a great deal about the signs of this disease. As the caregiver for a very wealthy woman, my first patient with this disease, I read articles about it and asked questions, but my experience with her taught me a lot. I lived in with her in her apartment on Lakeshore Drive in Chicago, IL, five days a week. She was an elderly lady with one daughter and she was in the advanced stages. Zanex was one of the medications I was to give her daily and she was never to miss a dose. I did, however, forget to give it to her one day at the proper time and she became very difficult to deal with, and I didn't realize it was because I had missed giving her the medication, which kept her calm.

The first few days I took care of her I was fine and I wanted very much to help her, but she was past that and as more and more time passed, my being there with her began to affect me. Now you may say it would affect anyone or drive you crazy living with someone with Alzheimer's 24 hours a day, 5 days a week, but mine was a different situation since I also had this disease, but not in the advanced stages. She didn't recognize me as the lady who had been taking care of her for quite a while, but what affected me the most was the fact that she didn't remember that her husband had passed away. So each day when we sat down for dinner she would ask me if he would be home for dinner, when I would tell her he had passed away.She would say, "No, he didn't." I was with her for about a year and this went on every day until I dreaded dinnertime and it began to affect me mentally; I felt like someone was picking at my brain and it seemed as though I was about to go insane, like I was being tortured mentally. It took every ounce of strength I had to survive during those months.

Florence Walker

I can understand how prisoners of war are broken down after being subjected to the same kind of torture hour after hour, day after day, only they are not allowed to rest. It was at night when I went to bed and on weekends when I was off work and went home that I was allowed to rest. Finally I was taken off that case. Sometimes when this woman would repeat the same question to me, I felt like covering my ears and screaming, but by faith I endured this also.

With each patient I took care of after that, that was stricken with this disease, I knew the symptoms, and was able to help one family that was unaware their father had Alzheimer's. After taking care of him a few days, I told them of my suspicions, after which they took him to a doctor and he was diagnosed with this disease. He was, however, far advanced, for he didn't even recognize his own home and asked every day to be let out of the house so he could go home. We kept the door locked so he couldn't go outside by himself. Not long after he was diagnosed, his family put him in a nursing home. I knew this was necessary, but I hated to see it happen because I knew of the physical abuse that took place in those facilities. In all of this I never recognized the symptoms I had; I couldn't help myself. But the time, God's time for my deliverance, hadn't come for me.

Oh, how thankful I am as I remember those I took care of with this disease, and when I see others today stricken with it (my own husband being one of them) that the Lord did not (it was not part of His plan) allow me to live or be tormented any longer by this disease than He did. I still volunteer my services at both a nursing home and a retirement home for seniors and both these establishments have units for Alzheimer's patients. Some don't know they're in this world; others are so confused they don't know their own families (this I learned firsthand as I talked with one, not knowing at first she had this disease); they cry and reach out to you as you go by. I feel so sorry for these poor souls and I pray and ask God to have mercy on them. He has shown me such great mercy, for I could be in the same state they are and every time it comes to me, I thank Jesus Christ for healing me.

Florence Walker

Chapter Seven

HOPE AT LAST

There is a stigma amongst the people of God concerning this disease a well as others and it is needless. It's a shame because it's a terrible debilitating sickness that is terminal. No one has the say-so as to if they will have it or not.- rich or poor, whatever we are in life. As we well know, if this were so, none of us would have it. Some of you reading this book will find down the road that you have been stricken with it also. It goes unnoticed for many years. The powerful, the famous, young and old; it knows no colors or nationalities, no one is exempt from getting this disease; and only those who have faith and trust in Jesus Christ can be delivered, healed and made whole from it. It is no different from cancer, diabetes, multiple sclerosis, and other terrible diseases to name a few, so why the stigma?

Recently I talked to the daughter of someone I have known for many years. Her mother has the symptoms of Alzheimer's, which I discovered after working with her for about a month. I don't know if she has it, only a doctor can tell for sure, but she has the signs. She is in her early seventies and has suffered two minor strokes in the past. I called her daughter, whom I've known since she was a teenager, to tell her of my suspicions and to suggest that she take her to the doctor to be evaluated.

Well, I'm sorry to say that she was offended by what I said. I explained that I was only trying to help her so that if she had the disease she could be healed (these people believe in divine healing), but she refused to even consider taking her to a doctor, saying that she didn't have Alzheimer's. She didn't have an explanation for things I told her I had seen; she was very adamant and upset. This was very foolish because her mother is the one who will go through unnecessary suffering, not her, and even if they didn't have faith to be healed, there is one particular medicine that I know for certain helps people, not all, stricken with this disease and that is Aricept. I have seen this for myself. Why allow your loved ones to suffer just for foolish pride? I hope and pray that she will have a change of heart because she knows some of the symptoms her mother is showing to be like Alzheimer's, but refuses to consider it even though she herself is a certified nurse's aide.

During all the years I suffered with this disease not knowing I had it, but wondering what was wrong with me and what was happening to me, I wanted help. I waited, hoped for and watched for my help to come during the time each episode took place, because in between these episodes I'd forget what had happened to me. I would have welcomed any suggestions given me to end my torment. Then, near the end of the year 2001, I learned that I had Alzheimer's. Immediately after learning this, I realized and understood the reason why all the things that had happened to me over the years had happened. I had been doing some of the same things the people whom I took care of were doing. I finally knew what was wrong with me.

I was so happy and felt such great relief. Yes, this was a terrible, devastating and incurable disease (as far as man is concerned) but I now knew what was wrong and I knew what to do about it because as soon as I got to church I was going to get prayer to be healed. We have healing services at my church and prayer is offered at every service. I waited until that Sunday, and when my pastor, Rev. Aleta Burnett, called for those who were sick to get prayer, needless to say, dear reader, I made it my business to be the first one in line. I told her what I wanted her to pray for. As she began to pray, I felt something happen in my head. I can't explain what it was, there are no words I know to explain it, but there was definitely something that happened to me and I was healed right then. The best way I can describe it is that it was like I felt many small things moving around in my brain.

If there was ever a time that I believed God, I believed Him then because He was my only hope; Jesus was my only help. This was the time He had planned for my healing. I no longer had to suffer, be confused or tormented; this was His time for it all to end for me. Oh, how grateful I am as I write these words. I'm also grateful for the experience I had and that He only allowed me to go just so far before healing me. This was done so that I would be a witness for Jesus Christ, to His great and awesome healing power. Oh, how happy and relieved I am to be free of all that I went through. Although I am glad to be a witness for Him, I would never want to go through the suffering and mental anguish I went through again, and hope that it's not His will that I do, or anything similar to that, either.

In 1988 my pastor encouraged me to go back to school to get my GED, so I started attending evening classes in Phoenix, IL. This was an extremely difficult task for me since I couldn't focus or remember things from one moment to the next and I really didn't even want to think of trying to learn anything again with my thinking being so messed up. It was all I could do to remember old things, but I went and passed my tests and was so proud and happy! Not only did I pass my tests; I was asked to represent my class at the graduation. Of course I was very reluctant to do this because of my mental state; I was so afraid of what might come out of my mouth without my meaning to. But again, my pastor encouraged me to do it. This was something that took prayer and a lot of courage as well as faith on my part. I really had to trust the Lord to help me because I didn't know what I would be faced with.

This was such an honor for me; nothing like this had ever happened to me in my life. There were so many people there to see me graduate, and this was unexpected because when I graduated from grade school no one was there for me. My mother had to work and couldn't afford to miss a day because we needed the money. I tried to understand, but no one came to see me. But, dear reader, when I graduated this time, I felt so honored. My mother was there, for which I was so grateful and happy even at the age I was - not only she but my two younger children were there (my oldest was ill and unable to come), my pastor, our bishop, my adopted mother as well as my stepdaughter. I WAS SO HAPPY! It was a struggle for me, but it was well worth it. Not only that, but as we went to change our robes, a young woman came to me and told me how much I had encouraged and helped her with the speech I had given. I was so very grateful to God to have blessed me to help someone else in the condition that I myself was in.

I prayed as to what I should say for a speech and the Lord gave me what to say. That young woman was proof of this. And then, dear reader, to top it all off my son surprised me with a graduation ring. I wanted one so much but couldn't afford it; he didn't have a lot of money but sacrificed to buy it for me and I cherish it with all my heart. This was just another experience in my life, albeit a good one, while stricken with this disease.

Now that I am healed, life is so much easier to live. Now I can be confident and sure of myself and don't have to wonder if I said something that was ridiculous or crazy or try to figure out if I understood correctly what has been spoken to me. Familiar words are not difficult for me to call to memory and more and more parts of my life that were lost and wiped out are gradually returning to me. It's no longer difficult for me to understand what's being said to me.

I am at the writing of this book getting ready to go to Bible college to get my degree (I'm 69) and I eagerly look forward to it, for this is a big step for me. A few months ago I got a job working at a high school in the media center. This was a new field for me because I had never worked on a computer before, let alone owned one, but I wanted to learn. My supervisor would give me assignments on the computer. While being trained, if I made a mistake I would ask the young lady training me not to tell me how to correct it because I wanted to figure it out by myself, and when she left me alone I was still able to figure out what to do and was so happy and excited because I knew what to do on my own.

Since I have been healed, I have gained great confidence in myself. I'm not saying everything has come together all at once; it hasn't. It took many years for me to get in the state I was in mentally and the progress I am making is gradual but not slow. I'm able, after not being able to for many years, to put things together. In my new found confidence, I believe that if there is something I want to do or need to do and someone else has done it before me, I can learn how to do it, too; all I need to find is the method. If it worked for them it will work for me, and I've had the opportunity to prove this. I can tell you, dear reader, I have never before had this attitude, never in my life. Before my attitude changed concerning my learning to work a computer, I never wanted to. It seemed too complicated and difficult for me, and before the Lord healed me I wasn't ready for a mental challenge like this, but the girl on my job who trained me was a good teacher and a patient one; she, as I said before, helped me a great deal.

I am so proud of myself; I am learning and remembering again. I was just like a child on my job and had to restrain myself every time I was able to figure out something for myself. The girls at work were happy for me also. So, I began to look for challenges and ask for new assignments on my job. Now, I love challenging work and I can tell you this is a first for me also. I still don't know a lot about computers, only the basics because they couldn't teach me that at work, but they have opened up a door for me and I have been blessed with a computer of my own so I can practice at home when I have the time.

Do I forget things now? I sure do, but not continuously and not without remembering what I forgot because it comes back to me. Things are no longer lost to me mentally; when I misplace something, I can recall where I put it. There is one exception, though. I have put my sewing machine pedal away and I still don't remember where it is, but I know it will come to me. Maybe now that I've written about it I'll recall where I put it.

I've taken a number of trips with my husband, following trip plans to South Carolina, Mississippi, North Carolina, the Wisconsin Dells and other places and I drove myself. I did get turned around a couple of times, but it wasn't a catastrophe for me as it was before. I wasn't shaken up; I found my way and kept going. Did I get nervous? Yes, but I was okay and not confused. I no longer get mixed up and unable to focus. Do I wake up sometimes wondering what day it is and where I am? Sure do, but it's no longer a problem because I immediately remember where I am and what day it is. I no longer live in terror, I'm happy and at peace. I am no longer tormented because of Alzheimer's disease and this alone means so much to me.

If I could only tell you and express to you, dear reader, how I feel now that I'm healed and delivered. I'm getting my life back. I hope that I find out before the Lord calls me home what kind of person I would have been if this disease hadn't robbed me of so many years. But, if I don't, I am pleased with the change in my life and thankful that Jesus Christ is not dead and that it was He and He alone that healed me and made me whole. I'm no longer the miserable, sick, tormented and unhappy person that I was. I thank God for Jesus Christ.

I'm grateful for those who were placed in my life: Rev. Jeannett Butler, Rev. Aleta Burnett and the late Bishop Stan McCurty, who were strong pillars in my life and who God (I now know) used to sustain and help me in spite of my not knowing what was wrong with me. It was their life, strength and prayers that helped and encouraged me to go as far as I did. My children, whose love I've had, if not always their patience, were a comfort to me. I sincerely hope and pray that this book will find its way into the hands of those whose loved ones are manifesting the symptoms of this disease and that they will take action to help them. Please don't passively sit by and do nothing. Don't be ashamed. They can be helped; they can be healed. I appeal to you on their behalf for they cannot. Take them to be diagnosed by a doctor.

As I said before, if you don't believe in healing, there is medication that will greatly help them, if only for a little while. Don't allow them to suffer any longer from this disease and, please, I know that it requires a tremendous amount of patience on your part, but THEY ARE REACHING OUT TO YOU IN THEIR OWN WAY FOR HELP. Trust me, I know. Don't speak harshly to them, don't turn a deaf ear to them because they are elderly and chalk it up to age. Don't treat them as though they are crazy, YOU ARE THEIR FAMILY AND THEY NEED YOUR HELP AND UNDERSTANDING. If you're not there for them who else will be? If you don't love them, who will? Remember, YOU MAY ALREADY HAVE THIS DISEASE YOURSELF.

I hope that this book will cause you to trust and have faith in Jesus Christ, not only to be healed of Alzheimer's, but from any sickness or disease. This is for real; this is for today. With his (Jesus') stripes we were healed (Isaiah 53:5). This is for you no matter who you are, if you want it. There is no discrimination, there are no special ones; the invitation is for all people everywhere, for all time. Come to Him and be healed and made whole.

Evangelist Florence Walker is available for speaking engagements and personal appearances. For more information contact:

**Florence Walker
C/O Advantage Books
P.O. Box 160847
Altamonte Springs, Florida   32716**

To purchase additional copies of this book or other books published by Advantage Books call our toll free order number at:
1-888-383-3110 (Book Orders Only)

or visit our bookstore website at:
www.advbookstore.com

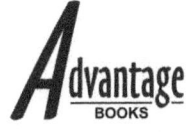

Longwood, Florida, USA
"we bring dreams to life"™
www.advbooks.com

www.ingramcontent.com/pod-product-compliance
Lightning Source LLC
Chambersburg PA
CBHW020021050426
42450CB00005B/591